Insensit

By: Joey Lew

Insensible Losses

By: Joey Lew

Nymeria Publishing, LLC

First published in the United States of America by
Nymeria Publishing LLC, 2024

Copyright © 2024 by Joey Lew

All rights reserved. Except as permitted under the U.S. Copyright Act of 1976, no part of this publication may be reproduced, distributed, or transmitted in any form or by any means, or stored in a database or retrieval system, without the prior written permission of the publisher.

Nymeria Publishing
PO Box 350747
Jacksonville, Fl 32235

Visit our website at www.nymeriapublishing.com

ISBN 9798988333296

Printed in U.S.A

For August, a constant source of joy

Table of Contents

I Want to Tell You That It Won't Happen to You, | 3

Sickness in the Time of Health | 4

Epileptic's Drug Cocktail | 6

My Parents Took Me on a Cruise as a Child | 7

Any Poem About My Body Is a Prayer | 9

I Chose California for Medical School Because They Don't Have Hurricanes | 10

Localization Exercise | 12

I Am at the Stage of My Medical Education Where I Only Know What Questions to Ask and Not How to Answer Them | 15

Remission | 17

Look: | 18

A Hallelujah for Triumph | 20

On an Organ Donation Run | 22

Some Babies Are Coneheads | 24

one summer i studied liver transplant | 26

Takotsubo Cardiomyopathy | 28

Overnight at the County Hospital | 29

Non-Maleficence | 32

Portrait of the Colorectal Surgeon as Echo | 33

Portrait of the Endocrine Surgeon as Gardener | 34

Hope | 36

This is My Self Care Poem | 38

Portrait of the Trauma Surgeon as Artist | 40

Portrait of the Trauma Surgeon as Atlas, Greek Titan | 42

We Live with Things that Hurt Us All the Time | 46

Portrait of the Minimally Invasive, Foregut, & General Surgeon as Oasis | 47

After Even Your Palliative Surgery Is Canceled | 49

Insensible Losses | 50

On Deciding to Become a Surgeon | 52

Portrait of the Pediatric Surgeon as Siberian Iris | 55

Holding Pattern | 57

Historic Storms | 59

The following poems have previously appeared elsewhere: Any Poem About My Body is a Prayer (*One*), one summer i studied liver transplant (*One*), Look: (*The Moth*), On an Organ Donation Run (*The Journal of Medical Humanities*), Overnight at The County Hospital (*Semicolon*), Portrait of the Colorectal Surgeon as Echo (*The MacGuffin*), Portrait of the Trauma Surgeon as Artist (*The MacGuffin*), Holding Pattern (*The MacGuffin*), We Live with Things that Hurt Us All the Time (*Free the Verse*), My Parents Took Me on a Cruise as a Child (*San Antonio Review*), and I Chose California for Medical School Because They Don't Have Hurricanes (*San Antonio Review*).

I Want to Tell You That It Won't Happen to You,

whatever it is. My first day
in the neuro-ICU I was
a patient. I will never forget
how small I felt under
thin sheets with an army
of professional gawkers.
There are no words for
the fear of post-ictal
paralysis. When I returned
as a medical student
my patient was intubated
and she looked just like me
and let me tell you I almost
lost it. All of it.
I want to tell you
it won't happen to you,
but then why
would it happen to me?
The world is a bright
and scary place,
terrifyingly sparkly.
A rainbow powder keg.
I wish I could swaddle you
all, but I can't. And swaddling
wrong really puts us
in a predicament:
hip problems, increased
risk of suffocation.
I can promise you only
it was never our fault.

Sickness in the Time of Health

I. At the Infusion Center

Your head feels like fall. An autumnal softness.

October has been ruined for two years now.
My IV's wheels creak and swivel on linoleum

and you sit beside me, sighing.
The nurse with the many-starred nametag

adjusts me, rag-doll-like, puppet thin, twirls my chair.
Your eyes, amber siphoned from the tallest trees,

fall slowly to my feet where you settle, a puddle of
witless love. If we cannot write odes to animals,

who is left?

II. Walking My Dog

If I say something out loud, assume it is to my therapist.
I have been silent some time now and even the leaves whisper—
you look so tired, by which they mean broken, as even their
fabric tears from root-spine and I am so alive in comparison,
but still they whisper; their commentary catches in my hair.

III. Applying to Medical School

I have been told that I
will not be discriminated
against because my illness
is physical. I have been told
not to disclose mental illness;
I have been told of the wellness
programs, the wellness, oh
all of the wellness
I am allowed only to have
if I come in holding my own—
take a penny leave a penny—
there are the minds of others
left checked at this invisible door.
If you need one for a day you can have it,
but only for a day, please, there is a waitlist.

Epileptic's Drug Cocktail

pink, blue, white,
Depakote, Vimpat, OnFi,
makes you sleepy,
buzz out of
habit, cold curious
spots in eyes,
tremor paralysis, and
left arm vibrations,
too awake, always
alone and waiting
to time and
interpret, remains alive.

My Parents Took Me on a Cruise as a Child

& I spent eight days vomiting in the cabin,
watched 48 hours of the TV show *House*
on DVD. I can still feel the boat's undulations
if I close my eyes tightly, like the prodrome
to a nightmare—so it's incredible
that I didn't remember the first episode:
a teacher by the chalkboard
her muscles tonic-clonic collapsing
to the floor in front of her students amazing
that even after collapsing in front of my
classmates trying to ask for help but unable
to speak I would still months
later pull up this pilot as if to rekindle
my love of medicine & snark on the long
long road to a medical degree & of course
see this woman's tongue immobilized
her muscles rigid then jerking then rigid
the way I would feel my own tongue
glued to my teeth my breathing
short & rapid would wonder how I could
ever watch someone experience the horror
of losing control entirely & have the strength
to intervene—in the ICU I had many
subsequent seizures & in the several days
that followed my stay I checked my chart—
a file marked: video. It was only a transcription,
though, my arm dislocating forwards
& then backwards with a violence
I do not remember. My head swiveling
side to side. This story is uncommon,

but the things we are afraid of
as doctors are the same:
the fear we will be discovered
as inadequate, the patients
who remind us of ourselves.

Any Poem About My Body Is a Prayer

Challah loaves braiding together
make double helixes fragile
tugging chromosomes together lacing
neatly, checking themselves for
deletions. Any mistake is
visible in the lattice-work, the stitching.

In the year of your lord (not mine):
the sleeper cells climb spines and set charges
on power lines. I like to think that I vibrate,
not seizure but seism.

My basket of synapses is staticky.
I hand them out—here hand
here face here thigh here neck
here neck here neck I am
      whiplashed and disorganized
speckled with
      bruises of my own
doing clumsy and reckless
with my   limbs as I am: here
missing B cells
      one unit down
hear my organs thank me
      smooth muscle taut pumping
          regularly thank you
hypothalamus thank you medulla oblongata
thank you neural tracts and absentia
for the year I have been no quake and all earth—

I Chose California for Medical School Because They Don't Have Hurricanes

My air conditioner sounds like
"rales"— the noise you hear in lungs
filled with fluid. The whole house
is in heart failure.

One roommate kindles new romance,
the other and I sit at our laptops
nursing long-distance love
against the backdrop of groaning wind
and encroaching fog—perfect weather
for self-pity.

In my first earthquake, the house
palpitates. I am anxious to know
that other people feel it too.
That the whole world is having this
seizure with me.

Slowly I am growing into this doubt.
How day to day I cannot control
anything. How medicine attracts
the most anxious and determined people
and tells them that they cannot know,
ever, all of the things
they might have hoped to.

The walls of my room are saturated
with anxiety. Encrusted with it.
They are a bright white which is the same color

as harsh, and as angry. If they rupture,
what will they let in?
What will they let out?

I can hear a throbbing sometimes
at night, and I think maybe the house
is dying. But it's just the dryer.

I close my eyes and this house closes
its eyes with me. Together we are
rocked to sleep.

Localization Exercise

For each of these scenarios, please find the individual's cause of injury

Case 1

A man enters your clinic
disheveled
unkempt his hair
sticks to his slick
scalp out loud he perseverates:
same word one thousand times

localize his injuries: is it the brain?
The brain stem? Maybe it's the time

his father left & didn't say I love
you not once maybe his father left
a scar let's image him imagine him
saying different words imagine
we cure him imagine we are so bold
as to believe a cure is what he wants

Case 2

The same man but now he is shaking
localize the shaking: his nervous
system or maybe a disturbance in the ions
in his blood or maybe the waiting room
is cold quick offer him a blanket quick
ask him his name does he know it

Case 3

The same man but now he's a woman
send her home

Case 4

The same woman but now she's pregnant
we have to save the baby quick
visualize the baby will the baby
soon be shaking or perseverating
did the baby's father say anything
where is the father the woman
doesn't know send the woman
home

Case 5

The baby is born and out comes
the first man fully formed & still
whispering his word: *please*
he just wants a place to be
away from the tidal wave
a cot to lie on until the blood
can be washed form his new-born
old man's face you apologize—
profusely—but you need the bed
for the woman in case 3
who came back on the brink
of death

For discussion:
Can you localize her wounds?

Physical Exam: Skin made of leather. 1000 micro-punctures. The abdomen hard & tender from a soon-to-be removed baby. Her pulse: the cadence of *Welcome to The Jungle*. Her eyes bright & brimming. She is singing to you of all her pain.

I Am at the Stage of My Medical Education Where I Only Know What Questions to Ask and Not How to Answer Them

My body has forgotten
how to weep.
When the insurance bill comes—
9,000 dollars—
it is for a clerical error on the part
of the hospital. Two tests ordered
instead of one, only one
insured. I am learning
the US healthcare system the way
a boulder learns moss.
I press on its ground
and am rewarded with inanity
and vitriol. I am in
No Apparent Distress.
I Process My Problem List:

Patient complains of paroxysmal
pre-syncope and cephalgia
concerning for recurrence
of autoimmune encephalitis.

I am having headaches and dizziness
and am afraid I am Sick again.

Patient complains of being robbed
blind by billing and ignored by
her physician and unable to handle stress

the way she used to—offer psych consult—

dismiss.

In every patient I can hear my voice
like a harmonizing whisper.
It says, *I trusted you*, it says,
I can't afford that, it says,
*I came here because this was
supposed to be the best.*

Remission

Breathless and the treadmill can't siphon
agita from the soul when the words
start spilling something like
secrets: I woke up to a twitching finger
folks who get fasciculations
are often unwell but for some it's
benign I count nine times in the last
two weeks that might have been seizures
but probably weren't but when have
probabilities ever soothed
such sharp numbers yet blurred
by estimation it's been four years
but I'm waking up still in the ICU
with a double-dislocated
shoulder still thinking about
the nurse Erin who walked me
around the unit who smiled and told
me about her weekend plans
so that I would remember weekends
would see time passing in the form
of hope maybe and now I have forgotten
weekends forgotten sleep for other
reasons I come home and smile
and hold the dog and am held
and am loved but still
the current courses and I feel it
and it knows my name

Look:

how you pretty yourself blue & tight-
tied like sparrows with amber twine
in sharp beaks, idyls & idols & excess
in your mimicry of birds always asking
mouth open in fear look how you tremble

> a slight tremor, moderate maybe
> hands extended & shaking the doctor
> grabs your head jerks it back & forth
> says focus on his nose says focus, focus on

the dog: a giant black egg indenting thin-threaded
couches paws tucked gently one over the other
& smelling of fritos his belly a sanctuary to bury
nose & mouth & eyes in to bury birds in
would he take you too if he grew & grew would he

> swallow, stick your tongue out, shrug
> your shoulders, repeat how it feels
> when the body betrays you like it betrayed
> your grandmother & her father like how

the plants by the sill are each named: the fiddle fig
Vanessa, the snake plant, Nathan, thick ribbed green
leaves reaching for orange afternoon sun & enrobed
elsewise in a cool darkness a life worth flowering
for & you stare at them, will them a life worth blooming

> in your prime & wondering if it matters
> that the world might end before you do

its aperture tightening you ask the doctor
& he doesn't know where else to look

A Hallelujah for Triumph

Clerkships: wandering wards with stethoscope
& pen light asking questions words like
allergies? easy, like *intubation?* hard
rounded tongue pressing against stiff
syllables this year is plagued by a lack of
information, foresight, wondering which nerve
exactly is protruding there & why the name
has buried itself beneath sternum instead
of sliding off the tongue every question
has an answer very few of which
are stored elsewise in my body or brain
& so a hallelujah for the time I, me,
this body, slid a diseased lung out of
human thorax, caught a mistake in the medical
record & reduced a patient's stroke risk,
faced off with an attending & earned
respect (after earning anger), sutured
shut a wide c-section incision & watched
the wound heal, brought my patient a poem
every day of her hospitalization, convinced a
terrified preeclamptic mother that her
blood pressure was not her fault,
convinced not one, not two, but three
hesitant adults to get the COVID vaccine,
showed up for every friend's birthday,
cleaned my home, did my laundry,
never wore the same pair of scrubs
more than two days in a row, ate
food, drank water, did not

give up. There are small failures
every day but this is not a poem
about that. There's a cramped black
box in my skull I am every so often
tempted to retreat to. A hallelujah
for the triumphs that sustain us,
that welcome us instead
into the light.

On an Organ Donation Run

I am asked to close   up
           (the body)
It is my very first operation

I never used to write from gut churning
I used to look life in its beady eyes
and juice all the gorgeous out of it
like strangling a monstrous fruit
with bare meaty hands made from

wrist-wringing and knuckle-cracking
in the back of a windowless classroom
asbestos lining the tight walls
I learned Spanish and then forgot it, learned
Spanish and then forgot
English and every word and now
I am looking at lungs inside a person
being removed from a person
and every word is forgotten

her family is praying for her soul outside
    make it pretty for the family
and every stitch is mis-
laid and corrected *slip*
the tail under the slick thread
and how do you make a pretty thing
with meaty hands inexperienced
in the body
       and its openings

and its closings
      and this place is so dark
so clean and my mind is so keen and so eager
if only I can do this right—

I never used to write about bodies and now
I close my eyes and open
an abdomen I could tell you every secret
the liver has but they would all be
lies I never learned how to close
myself up after injury

always seeping a little luxurious grief
and this person she figured
perhaps a professional might give her the
dignity of a job well done
but her knotted skin
is sallow and my knitting is a stitch
my grandmother never taught me
she was a psychiatrist
and when she died
she didn't recognize her doctor
I don't recognize
myself in scrubs so blue
and optimistic
so small and drowned in fabric
lady whose lungs we took away
I hope you'll forgive me you
taught my clumsy hands
a new prayer

Some Babies Are Coneheads

Filing cabinets—rows
and rows containing the facts
of existence: *some babies
are coneheads; we can replace
any organ with a machine
(temporarily) except
for the liver*
and a compiler
runs the code
to grow—a thin
stripe of blood vessel
shorn from the temple
laid atop the brain
will seek roots
yes! the head will
self-irrigate if given
the tools and children
infinitely adaptable
inflexible beings will
scream fever
sleep without eating
breathe from their
bellies, cannot
lie and cannot lay
still; the pearl of
wisdom I picked up
today is this:
you have to weigh
babies' diapers

to know how much
they drank and for poop
we use the metric
system no one knows
how heavy the truth
is some slips
in the cabinets are
red this baby has three
weeks to live but most
babies with her disease
die before day seven
horrible yes but how
incredible to triple your lifespan
today a boy went home
with his nurse who
adopted him
a little girl stared
into her first birthday
balloon the star in the center
was yellow and she held it
with wild eyes and open
mouth the very picture
of wonder I never knew
a child who didn't
deserve a parade

one summer i studied liver transplant

patients their most intimate
cells scraped across plates & analyzed.

a girl my age dies two weeks prior to my meeting her
chart, entering her data. she too was
on the cusp of grown-up, perhaps further

than i am with my plastic reflex hammer
& white coat that bunches at
the sleeves. i stay up all night & fly

on a tiny private jet to a hospital
in another town just to watch the liver
removed from a petite person so otherwise

whole. she is me-sized. we both have brown
hair & i wonder if her liver were not for some
reason good enough could they take mine

(if the tiny plane crashed & everyone
else survived) & i decide that i want to plug in
& out livers—the delicate art of time stopped

of keeping the body lived-in for long enough
to allow sacrifice—a life somewhere else
soon to lose cirrhotic and huge

liver the body suddenly with enough space
for all of its packages & the liver
starts working right away

pumping out toxins & clotting blood
& nodding to the duodenum
snug against its underbelly

the liver makes no excuses—
gets right to work.
but i am not the liver

of my medical school. at best,
i am the small intestine—

absorb, absorb, absorb

occasionally, secrete. but still
in the OR i hold suction in the abdomen
of the me-sized woman looking

unconvinced at her shriveled liver
& am assured it is decades
younger than its host & well-suited

to the saving of lives.
a liver does not ask
if it is enough.

Takotsubo Cardiomyopathy

A routine physical exam includes the measure of
blood pressure. The pounding rhythm of systolic
and diastolic—of opening and closing the heart
at the right moments. *You will learn to tell
what the human heart sounds like,* the doctor says to the white
coats. The sleeves inch upwards and the collar sits low as if to say
yes—all business now. I will learn how to hear every murmur
a chest has to proffer and I will offer a diagnosis—ill, well,
heavy. *You know you can die of a broken heart—metaphorically,
sort of,* a friend says. She means that there is a condition

in which one dies of sadness, usually
after a loved one has died. This is a fun fact from
the internet. It is not a satisfying diagnosis;
you will never know why the blood, finally, sits still.

Overnight at the County Hospital

pain in my left arm makes me think about
how women present with heart attacks
short of breath & heart pressed down into

vertebrae less bluster & falling off of
gurneys & more anxiety sweating
tension & ten out of twenty women

with heart attacks will leave still
chest heaving but without diagnosis
they say 90 minutes door to balloon

time & these women they just go home
I ask about this to a spine surgeon
trailing him past midnight in the cavernous

back hallways past staff-only signs
at the general hospital his long white coat
my pale blue scrubs he says *uh huh*

& what balloon is it we're talking about?
then later a small woman whimpers in the ER
new joint formed between slender wrist

& elbow is admonished for recklessly
getting hit by another car her car: totaled
her job: massage therapist & two tall

men stand over her like reapers
trying to be kind by setting bones & siphoning

her fear but it is bottomless the radiologist

points with a pen in the corner of
his dark office the pin is misplaced
too late to do it again & amid all of this

failure my left arm is hurting
I can get hypochondria from hearsay so
I'm saying facts over & over again like:

things are better than they used to be
& half of med school graduates
are women & never mind leaky

pipelines the wrist is sewn & if I go
into surgery I'll hold more than wrists
in my hands I am aching for the chance

to be more than a statistic but rolling
into 2 a.m. the residents say *why don't
you go home you've seen a thing or two*

so I do unwilling to be an obstacle
& in the uber home the driver asks
about me won't stop asking about me

& I watch the app the whole way
small blue car on small green map
because men just don't disappear

like women I let myself out at the corner
walk in & lock the door heart throbbing

palpitating we leave the hospital

& the night treats us just the same

Non-Maleficence

Plain woman with growling voice whose breathing
was the clanging of out-of-tune violin strings pulled together
in last-ditch calibration, I brought for you Dickinson
& Szymborska & Levine, whose amulets against nothing
were still better than nothing, & did not tell you
that I stopped the poems before the end, cut out
the sad parts, brought you only to flowering places.

Portrait of the Colorectal Surgeon as Echo
For Dr. Wick

She says *no cocaine for one week
before surgery*. She calls him.
She says *I'll call you again.* She says
no cocaine for one week when she calls
him and he promises. She calls
him and he doesn't pick up. She calls
him and he forgot his clinic appointment
and she says he has *a problem with showing
up*. So she calls him again with her calendar
up and says *what day do you want
the surgery. I can do the surgery whenever
you can come in.* And he picks a day and
she says *no cocaine before surgery*
to which he says one week. She calls
him and his name is melting butter.
Short-lived in her mouth. She calls
and he doesn't pick up. She puts him
on the calendar. She calls:
no cocaine one week before surgery.
He picks up. He shows up. He is rolled
back. He says thank you. He says thank you
thank you thank you. She removes
his tumor. She says thank you. She says
thank you, thank you, thank you.

Portrait of the Endocrine Surgeon as Gardener
For Dr. Gosnell

A woman believes she is warmer
than her friends, but *some folks are just sunflowers,*
and can't get enough heat

        the crescent moon of remaining windpipe
        compressed by the heavy lopsided bowtie
        of thyroid must be pruned, must be weeded,

told to get his affairs in order a man sought
a second opinion (hers) with more calloused hands,
was rewarded with years, built himself a house, remarried

        she tends to the salt of the earth, stem, stalk, and
        seed, asks after the lovely daughter and lively grandchildren,
        asks after fire season, the fog melting and returning

necklace of blue wooden beads and three stars
on each ear, for years she has cultivated,
watched and waited, eying the blight

        born into, borne by each bowtie plant, some into a vast
        desert, but *some folks are just roses* and can't help
        but bear children with sweetness and thorns,

three wedding rings have been lost in the dirt
during digging season, tied to her scrubs,
slipped onto a hair scrunchy, knotted into a necklace

      she didn't notice she'd grown a garden until a friend
      stopped by, noted all the plants, saw her hands on every
      wilted leaf, lifting gently, asked her how long, how long—

she sees to the generation of generations, the seeds
that need staking for growth, partners with the sole sliver
of moon to offer the most predictable tide

Hope

You were bright yellow
when I met you, your
bilirubin with no place
to go now a pigment
in your skin, the blockage
a handful of hard yellow stones
I still have a picture of on my iPhone—
you wanted to know how many
and how big and so I showed you.
After one month I became
desensitized. What it is to feel
at the mercy of another's pain control,
the order-writing and drug dispensing
and the checking in but once
or twice a day. Setback after setback.
The hollow of hope
departing. The morning a gown
is found undone and hair
unkempt and dried food
crusting chin. To will away
the gaze of others. It took a month
but you healed. One day lifting you
from stained sheets and walking
in place, the strain of your own
weight making of you a pendulum,
the journey could be seen
for its length. A friend asks
after hope—how acquired,
how sustained—I see then

he has not met you. How the body
is the master of its own toes.

This is My Self Care Poem

& I praise the wisdom of redwoods
that grow & grow until nothing
but sky confines them; how they feed
their tall bodies with the not enough
earth drink decade after decade
of soil-soaked water from insufficient
rain & remain wide & rough &
approachable. This is my redwood
poem, which every new Californian
gets by allotment. This is my
self-care poem, where the pinking of
otherwise green leaves & the pointy
pool noodles of potted plants
& the hummingbird who works harder
than I have ever worked & yet
is effortless rewards my awe with
joy. How will you make this
sustainable I am asked of
surgery for I am trying too hard.
Very little left sustains the red-
woods. It is not their ingenuity
that maintains their beauty
but the expectation of less.
An obvious metaphor.
I ask my therapist who says there is
no if. You become
what is needed or perish
in the effort. This is perhaps
not my self-care poem.

I haven't ever had time
for such indulgence. This is my
the world is burning poem,
the body cannot survive so many
sleepless nights but it will,
sustainability is a lie,
we destroy everything that we
love first and foremost ourselves,
the world is burning and
everyone asks: who will look
after the trees? And the trees
do not ask but continue.

Portrait of the Trauma Surgeon as Artist
For Dr. Plevin

From crash after crash flowed
broken hips and mangled limbs and
she squeezed the shoulder of a man
who might have died but did not.
He lost both legs. Cardboard splints
scooped the remains of each
to transport him, bone shards
everywhere. She talked to him.
Cut into his abdomen and took stock:
an absence of blood. In trauma he
is called a save. A man who might
have died but did not.

I remember most the feeling of legs
that have lost the shape of legs.
I remember second-most the sound
of her voice soothing him. How it seemed
a dirge at first but then mellifluous, kind.

I scrubbed the blood from each white shoe.
I went home. I called a friend and cried. A man lost
both his legs and could have died
but did not. The next day: clinic.

A man who had survived
eight holes in his intestine, ten in his colon,
six in his stomach, one bullet tearing
through and through the front of his chest.

A long scar carving his left from right;
he did not show up to follow-up
for a year. It is a miracle
made of her hands
that he is alive. Another man
stabbed through the heart, his
chest cut open so that the muscle
could be manually pumped
each squeeze distributing
the blood to his brain
alive by the art
of salvage. She holds

the hand of the man who
could have died and he asks
how bad is it? And she does not
lie. He has wide blue eyes, closes
them gently. His fingers are
icy. She says *listen*. She says
this is what we're going to do.

Portrait of the Trauma Surgeon as Atlas, Greek Titan
For Dr. Kornblith

I.
She introduces herself
to an open abdomen
a man awaiting closure
a feasibility trial of cold platelets
poured back into bleeding people
he is waking up

II.
Consider the following when extubating:

> *Mentation   Protection of the airway*
> *The ratio between oxygen in the blood and the oxygen flowing in*
> *Patency of the airway   Hemodynamic stability*

There was a reason
you put the tube in,
is it ready to come out?

III.
Trauma activation & forest green crocs propelling along
slick hospital floors

> *This city is 7 miles x 7 miles—the field is here we are the field*

The chest made into
a clamshell the IVs
a tangle of seaweed

IV.
The ringing in his ears
the Ketamine the Dilaudid
the Fentanyl the ED cocktail of

>*Sir you're going to be alright, can you hear me?*

delirium the thud of shorn shorts & belt
on the bloody floor

>*I do this every day. My whole life.*

In that moment her palm
holds his entire world

V.
>*And we're sure he didn't have a pulse?*

A scan slowly reveals a man born with
a reversal of organs, a left liver, a right heart

>*You realize the CPR was done on his lungs, right?*

concentric gold diamonds heavy her ears
her left knee crosses in front of her body & rests
on the mobile computer

VI.
Today is the day with no friendly
chest x-rays; she does not eat lunch
nor notice that she did not eat lunch.
She orders & reorders the appendices

& gallbladders, necrotizing infections

& bowel blockages, until every patient
has had their operation on this,
the month's meanest Monday;
She spots a little ditzel on the heart's
wall a possible breach
a man in need of a window
in his heart a release
of fluid so slides a tube
into his chest to ease
the pressure his stab wounds
still oozing she gently
reminds him—the bottom line:
This is a big deal, but I can handle it

VII
In the lab studying platelets
the small & sticky life-bringers
everybody bleeds but only some people
stop the question of invention:
can we cool them
when we infuse them do they
come together do they clot?
the chance to debrief
with a husband who speaks
the same language
over dinner he asks
about the stab wound did it
pierce the pericardial sac?

VIII.
When she met the woman
who held the world before her
the resemblance was striking

the way her work & her family
intermingled the pillars
she began to build
were ornate yet sturdy
(She, Atlas, at last relieved
by she, Hercules)

IX
the heart is unruptured & the patient
can go sutured & happy the patient
can go the patient can
live *there is no greater satisfaction*
even if it means in a sense
I never leave

We Live with Things that Hurt Us All the Time

A bright pink pimple with suppurative
comedone, an arthritic knee with years
left to further degrade, the decision to withdraw
life support. A stranger yelling, yelling.

I thought there would be something curative
in becoming sand-filled, punched-on,
creatively cleaved. Instead, my chest hurts.

A woman came into clinic today
because she can't get up hills like she used to.
Of course, she says, *I expected this.*

Portrait of the Minimally Invasive, Foregut, & General Surgeon as Oasis
For Dr. Kumar

Small child with joyful ball-kicking foot is again
kicking a ball between his mother's knees

as she details the pain, one finger tracing her liver's
edge trailing along her rib to mid-back,

Yes, the surgeon says, *I can help you*. In every room
lives a telephone within which are many voices,

every language. The hold music pours forward,
fills the room. *It's ok, we can wait*, the A

around her neck an homage to family, to the cakes
stacked and decorated at home, to the boys

who will grow knowing a woman to be a great
many things. Her hair has one streak of red.

She always uses a clipboard and the smallest number
of incisions. A man whose stomach

has pushed up, shoved under and through the diaphragm,
cannot eat without the nearby geyser of acid

and pain, is skinnier than she remembers. *Yes*, she says,
I can fix it. The surgeon's voice is hot tea with honey.

Her posture is the lone palm in all this sand. She offers

an appointment in one week, a known distance

between here and water. She wants pictures of this patient's
esophagus, seeks the bird's beak or small pouch

or unnatural erosion, a birdsong of harm and consequence.
She makes promises with unbroken eye-contact.

Every slot in her schedule is double-booked. But still, she asks
after the one who did not show up, asks if it's possible

to call them, to make sure that their absence
is not a question, that their wounds are thin lines, almost gone.

After Even Your Palliative Surgery Is Canceled
For Mr. B

Straw-colored, the belly-fluid's epithet
meant to mean yellow meant to mean
not bile, another humor, plasma
pushed through kissing cells spread
as by a pastor's palms now permissive
of liquid the cells sampled' simple answer:
cancer. You built buildings. I know this
because you noticed every uneven
mark of flooring the unsightly steaming
heating units painted beige and grey you said
they ran out of space for covering.
You, a planner, would pause before
careening forward a calm gentleness
in your swollen calves and the way
upon standing you swayed your lungs
soon to be heavy with fluid too
you said "I'm vertical" as in upright
as in a pillar a spire no man is a
building I wonder with what passion
you will leave us I never would have
known how rich your life if your
wife had not said of the seashells
you delight in the noticing
the spirals and notching
a collector of minutia
in the absence of time.

Insensible Losses

There have been so many this year.
So we sit on small plastic chairs
with wayward oval desks tucked sideways

and commiserate over every
individual we could not help.
A man who cannot wash his hands for lack

of clean water and so brings back the same
abscess repeatedly and asks why we
can't fix it; the man whose wife explains

that he used to cook for her every day
who does not understand this word
stroke who massages her husband's

feet and straightens the hem of his gown
though he cannot speak to or see her;
the forty-year-old with six siblings

who in rotating shifts learn he is dying
of inoperable pancreatic cancer;
I cannot mourn them I cannot explain

them how a woman looks when she
is afraid of water and so cannot shower
has lost her sense of time and place knows

only she wants to stay here in the county

hospital, forever; the child who has become
addicted to pulses of oxygen as her only

metric of control who yearns to leave—
in surgery we speak of insensible
losses, the water that evaporates

from an open abdomen or
full-thickness burn, but in these cases
at least we are capable of repletion.

On Deciding to Become a Surgeon

I am waging a war with my parts
like a tired machine who rebels
against their mechanic,
refuses the oil change,
will not have their odometer
ogled. So many doctors must
convince their mothers to get
colonoscopies. Women who likewise
will not look in the mirror for fear
of a changing mole, & I see
these women in myself, the not knowing
of non-stop self othering
the body set aside & the mind
freed to focus on the task at hand:
constant triage. Three patients with bleeds,
an acute abdomen, a request for Ativan, two small
bowel obstructions & a woman
who does not want surgery
at any cost. & I have seen residents
work miracles, from under a leaning tower
of tasks retrieve a kind smile & reveal
the notes to be done. Nurse practitioners
wielding wound vacs with one hand
write orders (legs splayed from patient
to computer) with the other & few are aware
of their magic multi-tasking & the intern—
praise be to the intern—
who has already seen & stitched
the bleeding wound & cried wolf

only where there is wolf, necrotizing infections
where there are necrotizing infections
in cellulitis' clothing. I have seen water blessed
to saline blessed to lactated ringers
hung faster than the one syllable of
please. I have borne witness
to miraculous recovery, the ventilator
removed despite weeks too weak
to swallow secretions & the infection
inadequately controlled still receding
by dint of the body's enormous reserve.
I have seen do not resuscitate
written for the first time
in an old woman's chart,
a woman whose hand I have held & belly
I have pressed (I among many).

I used to have seizures is a fact
most people don't know about me—
convulsive & devastating, resistant
to four medications, & then resolved
with the magic of a new medication
that stripped my body of its anti-body antibodies;
my right shoulder dislocated
forward & backward
over & over & it went unnoticed—
the pain was like a fire I could not place.
Smoke everywhere but too stuporous
to see the source, the shock-like pains
of plasmapheresis & nausea & wondering
if the blood all left my body
& came back what sort of superhero
would that make me.

& in the clinic as an almost-doctor
other doctors told me that folks with
autoimmune encephalitis are
brain damaged. I have worn vulnerability
under & over my scrubs
in all its sticky slickness.
There are no simple victories.
The patient that survives but cannot eat.
Cannot walk. Cannot speak. The patient that does not
survive. I am learning how to bleed
the lovely out of the labor. Yes,
the sleep deficit, which affects even machines.
Yes, the hunger. Yes, the thirst. Yes, also,
the immense caring unseen by almost anyone.
The ritual prayer of labs checked
over the bed of each patient.
A war that cannot always be won
with tactics but must at all costs be saved
from attrition. Medicine.
The small woman lying in bed who does not want
surgery & her obstructed bowel whining
its high-pitched cries & the hours of counseling & imaging
& the calling of family & the calling of an interpreter
& the decision made, finally, to cut.

Portrait of the Pediatric Surgeon as Siberian Iris
For Dr. Vu

Her left shoe is cocked from the heel, her knee
on the hard floor so that she and this child

can be face to face, can have this tiny moment.
The girl has never eaten solid food. She has a fear of salt

on her tongue. *Many paths were chosen for me.*
This path was my discovery. Zoom visits with

the stained back seat of a Honda Civic starring
fat baby in the lens of a
cellphone

camera. *Keep getting fat*, she advises.
She has two kids. They made everything better

and harder. How a stranger's child can have your son's name
and still disappear. *The surgeon does not always*

have to be the team's captain. She sketches
an intestine on the wax paper of the exam table.

Imagine you are flaying open a mountain.
She never adjusts her glasses. Does not have

any nervous tics. *In the OR you are your truest*
self. A maxim. *I never recommend surgery if I can*

help it. Another. The winter of her life
was also a time for growth. Not everything

froze. She learned to remove a tall
lobe of abnormal lung, to excise dead bowel

and reroute, all in the tiny landscape of
a fresh belly in a greedy world. She asks

a patient about fifth grade, leans in and smiles
with her teeth. In temperate climates the Siberian Iris

is grown as an ornamental plant, all tall stem
and violet-blue flowers. Some would say

this is its resilience going to waste. *When the child
sits alone they are establishing their independence.*

Her laugh is bright and light, like she is surprising even
herself. *There is nothing but this and my family.*

She presses her finger into the bellybutton of a small girl
with brown and yellow hair, confirms a small defect.

When she talks about the choices she has made
her eyebrows crinkle with joy.

Holding Pattern

Some days I just want to be wrapped around
my soft & sweet black lab like bacon around a date,

bake complicated brownies with whipped egg yolks
& work out slowly & meekly like the espresso

reached my liver too quickly & gave up. Glück's new collection is all about
dying. I woke up with my ankle twisted not remembering

any activity & I am 27 years old. This world like a spaceship
is hurtling toward uncertainty & I like a spaceship

have just enough fuel for the journey & nothing
extra. My husband kicks the snow to check its

consistency, steals my hat for his cold ears, & later
presses my cold palms against his face which has

overheated. These are the facts: when I try to crack
an egg one-handed little pieces of shell sneak into the batter;

my soft & sweet black lab is 9 years old & will die one day
just like Glück, even if he never thinks about it.

These are the figures: a stooped pine sapling & its heavy
icy burden, a shuttered storefront & the graffiti that is

its neighborhood love song, a single bluebird who didn't

get the memo. It is decision time & I am a spaceship,

enough fuel to return, yes, or to go twice
the distance, keep telling my stories to the emptiness

that is not empty at all, but filled with particles
I am assured we are on the verge of discovering.

Historic Storms

in San Francisco, the hills
sloping tarmacs into reservoirs,
an erosion of trust among
drivers, each weaving
to avoid standing water
& as the small patio attachment
of my apartment fills
like an unattended bathtub
& spills into the greenery
shrouding the unshielded
garage roof & the snowbanks
reach drought-defying heights
I am trying to make a commitment
to this city in her blue dress.
>*Am I gendering this city*
>*so that I can subjugate her?*

Seven years. The length of a
surgical residency.
>*three to open & four to close?*
>*one to open & close & six to know when & where & how?*

I hear that children like swimming pools.
I hear this from me, twenty years ago,
my hands pruned & the tight elastic
strap of goggles red-lining my under-eyes.

You could swim in the San Francisco streets
this week. Some folks are kayaking
around their belongings
asking the buoyancy
of each book & heirloom.

This city has held me in his arms
as the shoulders I have stood on
have fallen away.
     Am I gendering this city
        so that I can feel both distressed & damsel?
I have been learning the art
of leaving which like losing
is easy to master. In the interviews
I give this information freely:
I plan to have children. Even though
swimming pools smell of urine
& Chlorine universally.

My dog detests wetness, how his fur
becomes dense & his ears
infiltrated by slickness. At the end
of her notes on the politics
of location Adrienne Rich says
"This is the end." She says
"This is not an ending."

My husband & I were
married at the ornate courthouse
here underneath a Christmas tree
despite my Judaism & it was
beautiful. The weather
was tamer then; it mattered
less where we were
& why we were there.

Acknowledgments

This book was the product of five years of observation and medical education and persistent neuroticism and joy. Gratitude is owed to many, first and foremost my husband, William Xu, who makes possible everything and then afterward more. My family, endlessly supportive and thoughtful—Dad, Mom, Alex, Daben, Jing, Denise, and Michael, thank you. And the British contingent who without fail cheers from afar—Papa Arieh, Teresa, Dina, Tim, and Ben. A thank you to my MFA cohort and especially to Wesley Sexton, Michael Pittard, and Jabar Boykin, who read and critiqued an early draft, workshop with me regularly, and to whom I turn for literary inspiration, wisdom, and whimsy. To my other two early readers who double as therapists, life coaches, drinking buddies, adventurers, twin souls: Bear Aragon and Kate Oksas. To other writers and phenomenal friends that have been honest and supportive, helped me parse the contract and make sense of this wonderful opportunity: Emily Morris, Evan Fackler, and Kris Brunelli. To Emilia Phillips, who taught me so much of what I know about reading and writing poetry, and J.D. McClatchy and Peter Cole who came before them in honing and shaping my poetic sensibilities. To all of the surgeons at UCSF who participated in A Woman's Cut, my poetic portraiture project: Dr. Plevin, Dr. Kornblith, Dr. Kumar, Dr. Vu, Dr. Wick, Dr. Finlayson, Dr. Ascher, Dr. Feng, Dr. Sosa, Dr. Gosnell, Dr. Mukhtar, and Dr. Kirkwood, and to Dr. Louise Aronson, my mentor for that project and in life. To the patients who have inspired, motivated, and taught me. Thank you to Nymeria Publishing, Kennedy and Sarah, for partnering with me through every step of this process and for giving this collection a home. To UNCG and the MFA program there without which the world would be undoubtedly sadder and less literary. And finally to Duke Surgery (and especially Dr. Migaly, Dr. Tracy, and Dr. Kirk), for seeing my poetic pursuits as an asset and not a diversion, and for taking a chance on me.

A quick note on two poems:
"Amulets against nothing," a phrase used in "Non-Maleficence," is a nod to and taken from Phillip Levine's "Inheritance"
"Holding Pattern" was written prior to Louise Glück's passing. I have long admired her work and return to it often.

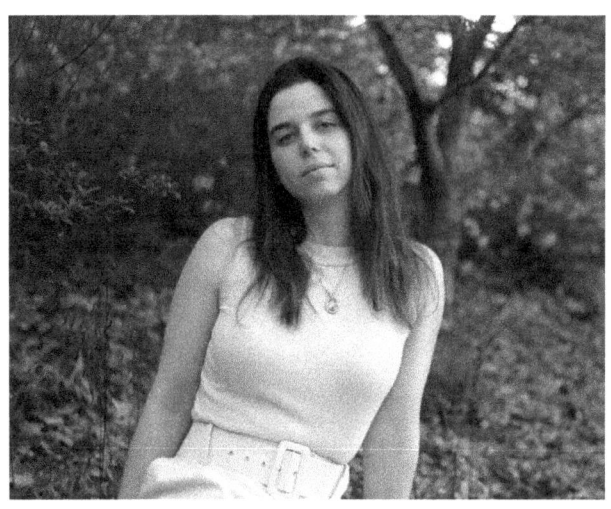

Joey Lew holds an MFA in poetry from UNCG and an MD from UCSF, and is currently a surgical resident at Duke. She placed first in the 2020 William Carlos Williams National Poetry Competition and the 2022 Lough Mask Poetry Competition, was shortlisted at the 2023 Wolverhampton Literary Festival Poetry Competition and was nominated for a 2024 Pushcart Prize. Her work can be seen in a number of literary magazines including most recently The MacGuffin and The San Antonio Review. This is her first book.

Printed in the USA
CPSIA information can be obtained
at www.ICGtesting.com
CBHW062122211024
16047CB00026B/836

9 798988 333296